A thoughtful guide for <u>anyone</u> new to drinking

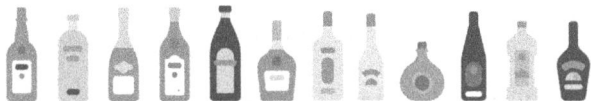

SAFE

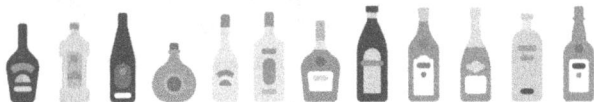

DRINKING

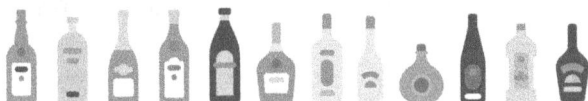

ACADEMY

HOW TO ENJOY ALCOHOL
WITHOUT HURTING YOURSELF OR OTHERS

MICHAEL HEALY

All inquiries should be addressed to Michael Healy
P.O. Box 1446, Shelton, WA 98584
Visit our Website at www.safedrinkingacademy.com

Design by Vanessa Mendozzi
I would like to acknowledge and give thanks to
Nancy Osa for her help in shaping and editing this book.

ISBN paperback: 978-0-578-71881-1

Library of Congress Control Number: 2020912822

CONTENTS

NEW TO DRINKING? EDUCATION BEATS PROHIBITION

When you want to drive a car or shoot a gun, what's the first thing you do? You learn how. You take a test. You get a license. Now, consider the first time you took a drink of an alcoholic beverage—or, if you haven't had one yet, think about what other people your age do. If you're under 21, you might hide it. You might drink too much. You might get sick. Or, you might taste it, get a buzz, and take it easy with family or friends for the rest of the night. Which of these scenarios sound best to you?

Obviously, the last one is the way to go, but there's something else that will help you enjoy what you're drinking: **learning how.** Our society and drinking laws are skewed toward the first three scenarios. We tell people under 21 not to drink at all, so they've got to hide it if they do. Advertising and sporting events may preach moderation but actually encourage overimbibing.

1

And a lack of any sort of training can lead to getting sick or hurt from drinking too much, or drinking in the wrong situations. The upshot? That's no fun. And it could be downright dangerous.

Consuming alcoholic beverages *should* be enjoyable. In a long human history of making and sharing beer, wine, and spirits, pleasure has always been the goal. It's too bad that the result is often unhealthy or life threatening. When you're informed, it doesn't have to be. **This book can help you decide:**

- whether you should drink
- how to drink safely
- what your limits are

But there's more. Data show that people under age 21 will and do drink, regardless of legal restrictions. If you're interested in trying alcohol, how can you do so legally? A majority of U.S. states do allow underage drinking in certain circumstances. But these lawful exceptions are not widely known. Could you name them?

So, if, while drinking, you run afoul of the law, what happens? If you harm your health, what might happen then? Again, these facts are far from common knowledge. We're more likely to know the advertising slogans for beverage brands than the consequences for abusing alcohol. Why? When making important decisions, it's best to weigh the pros and cons. But forcing teenagers to drink in secret, with little factual information, takes away that opportunity. It denies the chance to learn *how* to drink, within healthy limits and to the greatest satisfaction. Demonizing underage drinking confuses a trial period with a lifelong habit. This book will help people skirt those obstacles and begin a real dialogue about why, whether, how, and when to drink.

Knowledge gives you power. The power of choice, reason, discourse, and learning. Who doesn't want to know more about an intriguing topic? Better to learn the facts and cultural context than whatever the commercial ads tell you. They're not exactly neutral. Their job, after all, is to sell *more* alcoholic beverages. Responsible manufacturers realize that promoting moderation in drinking helps keep their industry sustainable. Yet, they want to sell more, not less, so their advertising taps into viewers' emotions. You'll hear the mixed messaging of "drink responsibly" along with visuals that encourage endless partying. The truth exists somewhere in between. So, the goal of this book is to reduce the emotional and increase the rational side of decision making, when it comes to drinking.

I should know. As an adult who didn't start imbibing responsibly until the age of forty, I've had my ups and downs with alcohol. I went through what a lot of teenagers are going through right now. Then, when I finally decided to take the reins and guide myself toward safe and enjoyable drinking, I realized I didn't know how. No one had ever taught me things like, how much is considered "a drink"? What's the difference between beer, wine, and liquor? How can I drink enough to safely enjoy the effects of alcohol without harming myself or the people around me?

I embarked on a mission to educate myself, and then to educate my children. Why keep young people in the dark about a topic they are bound to wonder about, one that will likely touch their lives in some way—even if they never take a drink? I want young people, as well as older folks who still have questions about alcohol, to know the facts and consequences, so they can make informed decisions. Learning from the experience of others is valuable. And it beats making potentially life-threatening mistakes yourself.

* * *

When I was growing up, my father and some of our relatives were avid hunters. It's a familial tradition best based in respect for the land and wildlife, in which game is taken in moderation and what's killed is gratefully consumed. And it involves the skilled use of deadly weapons. From a young age, before I ever was allowed to touch a firearm, my family counseled me in gun safety: never point a weapon at another person, leave rifles unloaded when not in use but treat every gun as carefully as if it *were* loaded. These rules were drummed into me, so that when the time came for me to handle a gun, I knew what to do.

But even folks who know how to drive a car in theory aren't just handed the keys. My father took the time to get me started, help me practice, and supervise my shooting technique. He explained how to spot a target, how to sight on it, and how to make sure it was safe to pull the trigger. He made sure I knew how to take a bird or a deer humanely, and what to do if I erred. In short, he set me up for safety and success.

Because of this, we loved to hunt. Every year, we camped out with friends and family and spent a week or a weekend hunting pheasant and ducks. At holidays, we would cook and share the game we had taken, dressed, and frozen. The ability to hunt with firearms gave us excursions and traditions that we treasured.

By law, I had to take a hunter safety course and maintain a valid hunting license. I credit these requirements and my family's vigilance with our safety record. No one in my extended family has ever had a safety violation or injury caused by poor skills or handling.

But, tragically, I do know of folks who have—people who hurt innocent bystanders or caused animals' suffering through ignorance or lack of caution. What could have been a satisfying hobby and time of bonding with family and friends became, for them, a dangerous or deadly mistake that changed their lives forever.

I find that hunting and drinking alcoholic beverages have much in common. They both involve mastering potentially dangerous elements in the pursuit of pleasure and fulfillment. They can bring great joy, or great sorrow. And the outcome of both activities hinges on our preconceptions, our attitudes, and our level of education.

* * *

The challenge for readers is to choose to learn more about the benefits, risks, and effects of drinking before ever reaching the legal age, which as of this writing is still 21 across the United States. If you gain knowledge before you build expertise, you'll get a jump on the emotional biases that guide so many attitudes toward alcohol. Many of these come from our family history, advertisements, peer pressure, and personal desires that shouldn't really be the basis for our decisions.

And they are crucial decisions. Unfortunately, our national approach to drinking is to forbid it until people turn 21. By then, we may have already formed opinions and habits that are unhealthy, and that also prevent us from having a pleasant relationship with fortified beverages. As Gabrielle Glaser writes in the New York Times:

> The roots of this extreme drinking lie in our own history. Prohibition, which banned most alcohol in the United States from 1920 to 1933, normalized the frenzied sort of drinking that occurs today at college parties. In speakeasies, the goal was to drink as much

and as soon as possible, because you never knew when the feds would show up. Today's law, likewise, encourages young people to dodge the system. Like Prohibition ... it's *been* a dismal failure.[1]

Denial will not reduce the risks or eliminate the reality of underage drinking. It won't answer important questions that young people have. Raising the national legal age to buy and consume alcohol in 1984 was meant to prevent accidents and fatalities associated with underage drinking. But reforming driver education and licensing may *have* had as great, or better, an impact.

We'll address this conundrum and other issues surrounding youth and alcohol later in this book. Even if you're over 21, chances are you've never been formally presented with the relevant information. My goal is to present the medical, legal, and social facts that you need to know, preferably before you begin drinking, and definitely in the event you already have. That's because, as with my own children, I trust you to make

---

1 Gabrielle Glaser, "Return the Drinking Age to 18, and Enforce It," *New York Times*, updated February 10, 2015, accessed April 24, 2020, https://www.nytimes.com/roomfordebate/2015/02/10/you-must-be-21-to-drink/return-the-drinking-age-to-18-and-enforce-it.

your own choices. But you can't do that without the knowledge and context that will help you thoughtfully consider the subject.

There's one more thing: **I believe learning and growing should be fun.** Like the culture of marksmanship and game hunting, the history, information, and context surrounding alcohol are fascinating. The act of sipping a drink is liberating, bonding, and satisfying. It may not be for everybody. But it's up to you to decide.

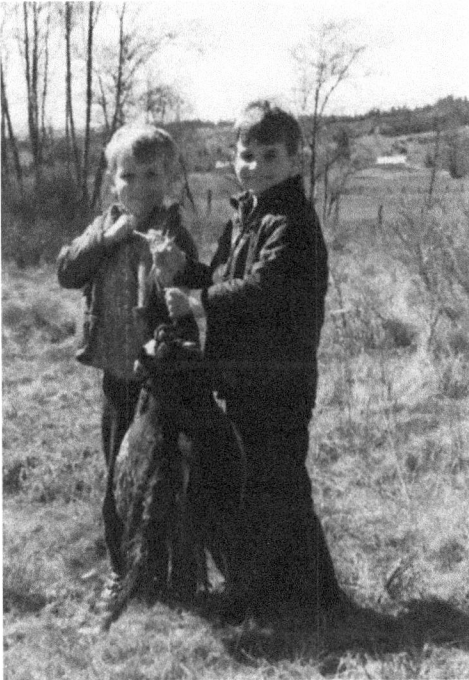

1

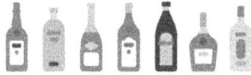

HOW DID WE GET HERE?

A Brief History of Alcohol

So many rules and regulations surround drinking that we may
forget alcoholic beverages, or their equivalents, exist in nature.
Certain strains of bacteria and fungi such as yeast can ferment
fruit. These microorganisms turn some of the sugar in fruit into
ethanol, a chemical compound known as simple alcohol—
which is intoxicating when ingested. Animals were likely the
first to eat or slurp soft, fermented fruit in the course of foraging.
Who knows whether they connected it with feeling woozy and
either sought it out or avoided it after their first "drink"?

Ethanol: a colorless volatile flammable liquid C_2H_5OH that is the intoxicating agent in liquors[2]

But, later, humans did. And some of them concluded that intoxication was a good thing, so they learned to make their own fermented drinks. Archaeologists have determined that these may have been kept in clay jugs as early as 10,000 BC, with evidence that wheat and barley were used to make beer around that time, in what is now known as the Middle East. Winemaking came later, in Asia, about 7,000 BC. By the rise of the Roman Empire (27 BC onward), wine's popularity had spread through Western Africa and Eastern Europe to the Mediterranean region. Although fresh water was in good supply in Ancient Rome, wine was considered so necessary to daily life that everyone, from slaves to emperors, drank it.

Liquor—such as whiskey, rum, gin, and vodka—is a purified, or distilled, form of fermented liquids that give them a higher alcohol content than beer and wine. The process of distillation was first applied to making perfumes, and may have been used

---

2 Note that all terminology definitions are from Merriam-Webster Online Dictionary, accessed June 6, 2020, https://www.merriam-webster.com/.

to produce a weak liquor around the time of the Roman Empire.

So, mammals have ingested and, perhaps, enjoyed the intoxicating effects of alcohol throughout history. A deeper understanding of those effects has developed in the past two thousand years. We now understand how humans **metabolize**, or physically process, the alcohol we drink in beverage form. We know how it affects the human body, in good and bad ways, and in adolescence versus maturity. How drinking alcohol affects the mind is a subject of greater disagreement, one clouded by emotional, political, and religious motivations.

Metabolize: to subject to metabolism, or the processes by which a particular substance is handled in the living body

For instance, alcohol consumption has been blamed for social problems like crime, poverty, and poor work habits, although these have many complex origins. On the other hand, alcohol has been used to motivate laborers, as it was during the 16th through 18th centuries by the English navy and army. It has also substituted for daily water rations, when typical European water supplies were tainted by sewage and debris. In 1620 when the English ship *Mayflower* set sail for the New

World, for example, it carried more barrels of beer than of water. Since fermentation killed harmful bacteria and preserved the water content of beer (93 percent by weight)—and because beer contains some vitamins, minerals, and caloric energy—it was considered a valuable dietary staple. Its intoxicating effects were seen as either a bonus or a detriment, depending on the prevailing attitude or conditions.

Alcohol consumption, then, has been a part of North American culture since before our nation's inception. The social acceptance of drinking in general, and drinking by young people in particular, has changed over time. Let's look at how those views came about.

A Timeline of Alcohol in America

1700s: Local governments impose license requirements to sell alcohol and fines for public drunkenness. Religious groups and civic leaders begin to call for people to curb drinking for moral and health reasons.

1800s: Industrial Revolution demand for productive workers causes attitudes about drunkenness to change.

Negative views of drinking lead to an organized Temperance Movement promoting moderation in or abstinence from drinking. Industrial "company towns" such as Pullman, Illinois, are constructed to house workers and isolate them, with the intent of keeping them away from alcohol, improving their moral fiber, and making them more productive.

1900s: Temperance Movement rhetoric moved toward total abstinence from alcohol, leading to passage of the 18th Amendment in 1920 prohibiting the manufacture and delivery of alcohol. (Note that consumption was never illegal!) The 21st Amendment repealed Prohibition in 1933, after violent crime associated with black-market alcohol sales plus the need for new revenue during the Great Depression caused a change in attitudes toward regulation. In 1984, the National Minimum Drinking Age Act made 21 the legal age to purchase and possess alcohol in public, in all 50 states.

2000s: States begin to adopt graduated driver licensing for teenagers, with many jurisdictions requiring zero blood-alcohol levels to maintain driving privileges during a probationary period.

Pairing learning to drive with a restriction on alcohol consumption is a critical point, both for new drivers and for new drinkers. It points to the fact that people under age 21 *do* drink, and that impairment greatly increases risk for everybody on the road. The licensing rules also highlight that learning to drive requires adult supervision in every state, but learning to drink? That falls through the cracks. This don't-ask, don't-tell situation exists not just because teenagers, by nature, are exploring their boundaries and trying new things, which they may or may not want adults to know about. It's because, collectively, adults sidestep responsibility for teaching adolescents about alcohol, instead substituting prohibition for education.

Does that work? Statistics say, no.

Youth and Drinking

Despite a legal drinking age of 21, people between the ages of 12 and 20 are responsible for 11 percent of total alcohol consumption in the United States.[3] A Centers for Disease Control and Prevention (CDC) study published in 2017 found that 30 percent of high school students surveyed had imbibed some amount of alcohol in the previous month. Nearly half of those who drank admitted to **binge drinking**, defined as four to five drinks within two hours or less.

» Going on a Bender

A normal rate of drinking, about one drink per 90 minutes, allows people to safely metabolize alcohol. **Binge drinking—consuming four to five drinks or more in two hours or less**—allows alcohol to build up in the bloodstream to the point of acute intoxication. Binge drinking is an abusive practice that can cause potentially fatal alcohol poisoning in the short term or lead to alcohol dependence over time.

Binge drinking is a problem because it can lead to alcohol poisoning, which we'll discuss later. But binge drinking exists,

---

3 Centers for Disease Control and Prevention, "Underage Drinking," updated January 3, 2020, accessed May 2, 2020, https://www.cdc.gov/alcohol/fact-sheets/underage-drinking.htm.

at least in part, because those under 21 may have to hide their actions or fit them into a small time frame due to legal restrictions or adult disapproval. Drinking heavily and swiftly can raise alcohol tolerance, a risk factor for dependence, or alcoholism, now widely called **alcohol use disorder**. The U.S. Surgeon General reports that *Americans ages 18 to 20 have the highest rate of alcohol dependence of any age group.*[4] Does that sound like "prohibition" is working?

» What Is Alcoholism?

Alcoholism, or **alcohol use disorder**, is a physical and mental state marked by at least two of these conditions:

- regularly drinking large quantities of alcohol over a long period of time
- difficulty reducing alcohol consumption
- spending much time and effort in acquiring and drinking alcohol

---

4 Office of the Surgeon General (US), National Institute on Alcohol Abuse and Alcoholism (US), Substance Abuse and Mental Health Services Administration (US), *The Surgeon General's Call to Action To Prevent and Reduce Underage Drinking.* Rockville (MD): Office of the Surgeon General (US); 2007. Available from: https://www.ncbi.nlm.nih.gov/books/NBK44360/.

- the desire for alcohol is strong and difficult to resist
- drinking interferes with the fulfillment of responsibilities
- intoxication results in social, health, or safety problems
- lack of alcohol produces withdrawal symptoms such as shaking or sweating
- alcohol tolerance grows over time

Certainly, the goal of preventing disease, death, and injury to others by using laws to curtail drinking—particularly by maturing individuals—is a good one. But laws that don't achieve that goal only generate contempt. We'll get to the physical risks and benefits for new drinkers in Chapter 3, and the legal ramifications in Chapter 4. Until the legal system finds a better solution, though, the alternative to reasoned consumption is education and practice under adult supervision.

That doesn't mean that every adult makes a great supervisor. They, after all, have grown up with something near the current model of initiation. They may have formed their own drinking habits without the benefit of relevant information. It's important to seek out role models whom you respect and trust. You don't have to drink *with* them, but you can learn from their example.

Self-education is your choice, but it may conflict with the viewpoints in your family or school. The most conservative views consider any amount of alcohol unacceptable. The most progressive may set no limits. **But you don't have to drink a drop to learn more about alcohol**. It's important to make that distinction. Even non-drinkers may one day find themselves in a situation where they need to assess whether a friend or family member has had too much to drink and how best to help them. And if you do wish to imbibe, the more you know, the better you can do so safely.

So, where do you fit in? How will your decisions affect your life? The lives of those you love? Now is the time to ask these questions, before your own views are set in stone. As you explore the possibilities, talk them over with people who have some experience. A dialogue may shed light on issues that are not clear-cut. Meanwhile, the following chapters will help you look more closely at:

- the different types of alcoholic beverages
- how these are produced and marketed
- how to find the right limits for you

- the legal consequences of underage drinking, and drinking and driving
- how best to enjoy alcohol—or how to confidently decline

Let's go!

2

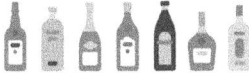

WHAT'S THE DIFFERENCE BETWEEN BEER AND ALE?

Hint: It's a trick question.

When you set out to tackle any subject, you've got to know the lingo. Drinking has its own terminology, plus more slang than any dictionary can contain. This complicates the process of selecting and buying alcoholic beverages, as well as drinking within your personal limits. For folks who choose not to drink, putting together a bar for company or finding the right wine for a holiday dinner can be challenging. So, let's delve into the terminology and related concepts that will help you make the right choices all around.

The most important term you need to know is **alcohol by**

volume, or **abv**. This is a standard measure of ethanol content based on the size of beverage container. Commercial beers, wines, and liquors may display their abvs on their labels.

In America, the alcohol content of liquor is also described as **proof**, which is twice the abv. For instance, vodka that is 40% abv is 80 proof. Why? Just to confuse us, maybe. This historical term that dates back to early taxation isn't really used for any purpose anymore.

The Wide World of Alcoholic Beverages, by Type

FERMENTED BEVERAGES

Beer. Beer is brewed from water and malted grains such as barley, wheat, and oats, usually flavored and preserved with **hops**, the flowers of an edible vine. Soaking and drying, or **malting**, grains creates enzymes needed to produce sugars and interact with yeast. The products of this process, called **fermentation**, are ethanol and carbonation—the alcohol content and fizziness that beer is known for.

Different ingredients and styles of brewing make different kinds of beer, such as **lager**, a lighter style, and **ale**, a more robust style. (To answer the trick question, ale is a type of beer.)

Today's craft brewers also use a wide range of natural flavoring agents, making raspberry, apricot, tangerine, and even pumpkin beers and ales possible. Beers range in color from very pale blonde (pilsners) to brown and nearly black (porters, stouts). Their alcohol content is usually between 4% and 14%.

Malt liquor is fortified beer that is more than 5% abv. **Light beer** has reduced alcohol content, typically no more than 4%, and so contains fewer calories. **Nonalcoholic beer** has had most of its abv removed, but still has trace amounts of about 0.05%.

Commercial beer is sold in cans and bottles or can be dispensed by the glass, pitcher, or "growler" from a large keg. Keg draws are called **draft beer**. Many small craft brewers without bottling facilities dispense beer exclusively this way. Take-home amounts may be poured into **growlers**, gallon-size jugs made especially for draft beer.

Wine. Wine is made from fermented grapes, or another fruit or grain such as plums or rice. Recall that fermentation occurs when microorganisms act on fruit to convert its sugar molecules into ethanol (alcohol). Winemakers take charge of this process to regulate the taste, color, and alcohol content of the final product. It begins with harvesting and crushing the grapes and concludes with aging in wood or stainless steel barrels to let the flavor develop. Wine is usually then packaged in bottles or pouches for distribution.

Grapes of different varieties determine the color and style of wine. **Red wines** are made from dark red or purple grapes processed with their skins. **White wines** are made from only the pulp of green or yellow grapes, without the skins. **Sparkling wines**, like champagne and prosecco, are made by trapping the carbon dioxide (CO_2) byproducts released during fermentation in the bottle. Regular, "still," wines are fermented instead in open-air vats to allow the CO_2 to evaporate. Finished wines usually have an abv of between 10% and 15%.

Wine **varietals** are the type of wine you'll see printed on labels. These are determined by the majority content of grape variety. You may recognize some of them:

- Cabernet sauvignon
- Chardonnay
- Merlot
- Pinot noir
- Zinfandel

The "brand" of wine that you'll also see on labels is the name chosen by the producer, often a family or vineyard name. The area in which the source grapes are grown is called an **appellation**. The year in which the grapes were harvested is called the **vintage**. Some or all of this information may appear on labels. (See a sample wine label later in this chapter.)

Cider and other flavored or malt beverages.

So, what about other commercially prepared, **"ready to drink" (RTD) beverages?** These are alcoholic solutions typically sold in single-serving cans or bottles. You may know RTDs as "hard" ciders, seltzers, teas, or lemonades, or by the brand names given to them by the beverage manufacturers that make them.

"Hard" cider is made from fermenting the juice pressed from apples or pears, sometimes flavored with other kinds of fruit. These can also be fermented in bottles to retain CO_2, for a fizzy beverage. Alcohol content varies, but is usually between 4% and 12% by volume.

"Hard" seltzers, teas, lemonades, or malt beverages other than beer vary widely in sugar and alcohol content. In addition to their base of fermented fruit or malt grains, these alcoholic drinks may be flavored with fruit or soda, sweetened with sugar, or even boosted with caffeine.

DISTILLED BEVERAGES

Liquor, **brandy**, and **liqueur**. Liquor (also known as **spirits**) is a beverage alcohol made from fermented vegetables, fruits, or grains that is stronger than beers and wines due to **distillation**, a process that reduces its water content. This increases the proportion of ethanol to produce a liquid that is 30% or more abv.

Popular types of liquor include whiskey, vodka, and rum, typically made from corn, potatoes, and sugarcane, respectively. These can be drunk "straight," with no additives, or blended into **cocktails**, which are mixed drinks made with liquor, fruit juice, soda, or other liquids. **Brandy** is a distilled wine, while **liqueur** (also known as cordial) is a liquor with enhanced sugar and flavoring such as oranges, mint, or coffee.

Distillation occurs in a **still**, a copper or copper-lined vessel in which fermented liquids are purified to raise the alcohol content and control the flavor of the finished beverage. Heat is used to separate ethanol from water, because the two compounds have different boiling points. The boiling water evaporates, leaving the ethanol behind. Operating a still to make liquor requires a license in the United States, whereas making your own beer or wine does not.

* * *

That's a lot of information. We'll compare the experience and physical effects of drinking different classes of alcoholic beverages in the next chapter. But, to do that, you'll need to know what you're drinking at any given time. The laws regarding the sale of beverage alcohol require certain information to be on the product label. If you've learned to read the nutrition facts on packaged foods, you'll find these labels sorely lacking in details.

What they usually don't include is a list of ingredients and nutrients! In the case of beer, wine, and liquor, the nutrient content is low, but the calorie content is significant, in combination with the rest of your diet. Among other effects of drinking, weight gain is a factor you'll want to be aware of and avoid. But labels won't always help you do that. Ready-to-drink beverages, for instance, may be highly sweetened but aren't legally required to list a calorie content—while manufacturers of light beers are happy to offer up that information because fewer calories are their selling point.

For now, let's take a look at what alcoholic beverage labels *can* tell you ... and how to find what they don't.

How to Read a Label—and What Else to Consider

You've probably noticed the pretty colors of bottles or cans of alcoholic drinks and the graphic designs meant to create an image around each brand. Now, prepare to notice the more important packaging elements: the alcohol content and health warnings ... and also what is *not* on the label.

Reading labels tends to raise more questions than it answers. That's because federal requirements are very sparse: the only mandatory information includes a standard health alert, and the percentage of alcohol content by volume (abv)—but that percentage is only required for distilled beverages and for wine with more than 14% abv. That's it. No calories. No ingredients. No serving sizes or total servings per container.

In a regulation-heavy country, alcoholic beverage labeling is a notable exception. Companies can put that additional information on a can or bottle, but they don't have to. The self-interest of industry lobbyists has maintained these labeling conditions since the end of Prohibition in the 20th century. Sure, you can obtain those facts on manufacturers' websites. But they may or may not be easy to find, understand, or compare with other beverage statistics.

For instance, only wines with *less than* 7% abv and beers that *don't contain* malted barley need to list the kind of nutrition facts you find on other packaged foods—but not the abv! This leaves consumers in the dark about the exact alcohol content of most beers, wines, and RTD beverages, and the resulting sugar and calorie loads that they carry. Only hard liquor containers have to list their contents' abv.

Confused? That's the point. Providing more information could steer people away from certain drinks. But if you've got access to a smartphone or computer, you can play detective to get the data you need to make informed choices. First: **the abv**. That number is what you need to know in order to gauge your consumption limit and plan accordingly how much to drink, over what period of time. And second: **the calorie and sugar counts**. Those will help you manage your weight or health conditions such as diabetes, if you drink.

HOW TO READ A WINE LABEL

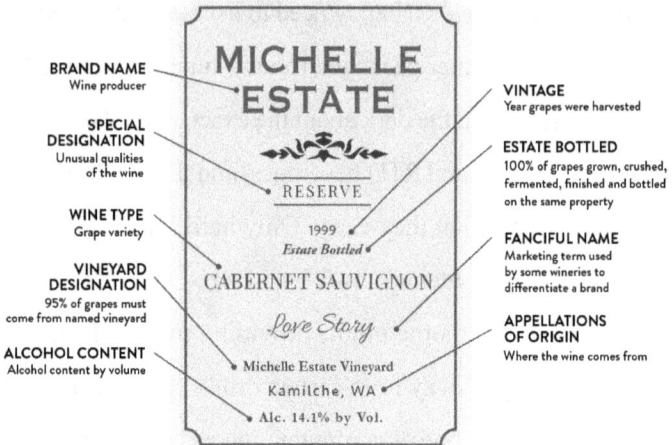

BRAND NAME
Wine producer

SPECIAL DESIGNATION
Unusual qualities of the wine

WINE TYPE
Grape variety

VINEYARD DESIGNATION
95% of grapes must come from named vineyard

ALCOHOL CONTENT
Alcohol content by volume

MICHELLE ESTATE

RESERVE

1999
Estate Bottled

CABERNET SAUVIGNON

Love Story

Michelle Estate Vineyard
Kamilche, WA
Alc. 14.1% by Vol.

VINTAGE
Year grapes were harvested

ESTATE BOTTLED
100% of grapes grown, crushed, fermented, finished and bottled on the same property

FANCIFUL NAME
Marketing term used by some wineries to differentiate a brand

APPELLATIONS OF ORIGIN
Where the wine comes from

What does the abv tell you about how drunk you could get? And whether you'll be able to safely drive or perform other functions? When taking into account your body weight and the amount of time you'll spend imbibing a drink, you'll arrive at your estimated **blood alcohol content (BAC).** This is the number that flashes on breathalyzer screens to tell the authorities whether you're past the legal limit to drive. **The legal BAC limit to drive in the United States is 0.08%.** Whether you're driving or not, if you're past that limit, you're on your way to being drunk, not just buzzed or tipsy. It's this state of intoxication that dramatically raises your risk for alcohol's negative side effects.

STANDARD SERVING SIZES

BEER	WINE	DISTILLED LIQUOR
12 ounces	5 ounces	1.5 ounces

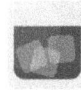

To determine your BAC, you can purchase a handheld breathalyzer or downloadable smartphone app from medical suppliers, or use an online tool, such as Cleveland Clinic's BAC Calculator.[5] For a rough estimate, try this chart based on one provided by the University of Pittsburgh.[6] **Note how many drinks will put you past the .08 mark:**

---

5 Cleveland Clinic, "Calculate Your Blood Alcohol Content," health tool, accessed June 6, 2020, http://www.clevelandclinic.org/health/interactive/alcohol_calculator.asp.

6 University of Pittsburgh, "Alcohol Facts," accessed June 6, 2020, https://www.studentaffairs.pitt.edu/shs/education/alcohol/.

Blood Alcohol Content Estimator by Gender and Weight

FOR MALES

Body weight (lbs)	1 drink	2 drinks	3 drinks	4 drinks	5 drinks	6 drinks	7 drinks	8 drinks	9 drinks	10 drinks
100	.043	.087	.130	.174	.217	.261	.304	.348	.391	.435
125	.034	.069	.103	.139	.173	.209	.242	.278	.312	.346
150	.029	.058	.087	.116	.145	.174	.203	.232	.261	.290
175	.025	.050	.075	.100	.125	.150	.175	.200	.225	.250
200	.022	.043	.065	.087	.108	.130	.152	.174	.195	.217
225	.019	.039	.058	.078	.097	.117	.136	.156	.175	.198
250	.017	.035	.052	.070	.087	.105	.122	.139	.156	.173

FOR FEMALES

Body weight (lbs)	1 drink	2 drinks	3 drinks	4 drinks	5 drinks	6 drinks	7 drinks	8 drinks	9 drinks	10 drinks
100	.050	.101	.152	.203	.253	.304	.355	.406	.456	.507
125	.040	.080	.120	.162	.202	.244	.282	.324	.364	.404
150	.034	.068	.101	.135	.169	.203	.237	.271	.304	.338
175	.029	.058	.087	.117	.146	.175	.204	.233	.262	.292
200	.026	.050	.076	.101	.126	.152	.177	.203	.227	.253
225	.022	.045	.068	.091	.113	.136	.159	.182	.204	.227
250	.020	.041	.061	.082	.101	.122	.142	.162	.182	.202

** These charts are intended to provide a general guideline for you. Every person reacts differently to alcohol and additional aspects such as body composition, use of medication or other drugs, mood changes as well as metabolism should be factored

Effects of blood alcohol content on thinking, feeling and behavior:

Now that you know how to calculate BAC, see how alcohol affects your body at different levels.

0.02 – 0.03

Legal definition of intoxication in many states for people under 21 years of age (Note: in some states, it is 0%.) Few obvious effects: possible mild light headedness and mild relaxation; yet, automobile accidents are twice as likely to occur.

0.05 – 0.06%

Slight sedation; feelings of warmth, relaxation. exaggeration of emotion and behavior; slight decrease in reaction time and in fine-muscle coordination; impaired judgment about continued drinking.

0.08 %

Legal definition of intoxication in the United States for people 21 years and older.

0.10 – 0.12%

Euphoria; motor skills are markedly impaired; lack of
coordination and balance; memory and judgment are
markedly impaired; recognition of impairment is lost.

0.14 – 0.17%

Major impairment of all mental and physical functions; slurred speech, blurred vision, and loss of motor
skills control; difficulties in walking, talking, and
standing; severe deficits in judgment and perception.

0.20%

Feelings of numbness; all mental, physical, and sensory
functions are severely impaired; nausea and vomiting;
must have assistance standing or walking; risk of severe
injury from falls and accidents; increased risk of asphyx-
iation from choking on vomit; needs medical assistance.

0.30%

Severe intoxication; little comprehension of the envi-
ronment; loss of consciousness can occur; difficult to
arouse; needs hospitalization.

>0.40%

Comatose; absence of perception; death due to respiratory arrest is more likely.

We'll talk more about these effects in the next chapter. Note that the chart above is based on an *average* alcohol content, which is fairly standard for liquor but varies widely for beer and wine. You'll want to be able to adjust for actual higher or lower abv. So, when you pick up a can of beer, bottle of wine, or bottle of vodka, look for the alcohol content percentage (not proof) on the label. Learn to pour a standard serving plus any mixers you might want. Then aim to consume it over the course of about sixty to ninety minutes.

I know; it's a lot of math. But once you learn how to do it and run through it a few times, you'll begin to understand your personal physical response and how to set your own drinking limits. This will help you stay out of harm's way and avoid negative consequences. It will also guide you in what to do if a friend shows symptoms of extreme impairment.

We'll delve more deeply these things in the following chapters. But you are already armed with one important tool: **awareness**.

3

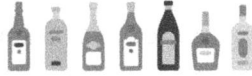

WHAT HAPPENS WHEN YOU DRINK?

The Good, the Bad, and the Ugly

The descriptions of the physical effects of intoxication at the end of Chapter 2 detail the immediate changes on the body, drink by drink. Most of the larger health repercussions, good and bad, occur over time. If you look forward to a long life of responsibly enjoying alcohol, then you've got to temper the downside of drinking. If you're in an ethnic or medically challenged group that has more severe reactions to intoxication, this is even more important—as is the question of whether to drink at all.

What actually happens when you drink? And what conditions affect how you, personally metabolize, or physically process, alcohol? Here's a quick description:

> Alcohol is a depressant of the central nervous system,
> which controls most functions of the body and mind.
> That's why it can be used as an anesthetic, and why
> drinking raises the risk for accidental injury and death: it
> leaves us less able to coordinate our thoughts and actions.

The effects of alcohol are based on its concentration in the body, which depends on the strength of a drink and how quickly it is absorbed into the bloodstream. We have seen the different strengths of different types of alcoholic beverages— such as beer versus liquor. This content can change when diluting drinks, such as adding seltzer water to wine or fruit juice or soda to liquor. In addition, the alcohol concentration in our bodies changes with the amount of food in our systems. For example, drinking on an empty stomach makes us absorb alcohol faster; drinking with or after a snack or meal slows the rate of absorption. Other factors that determine that rate are: the individual's level of body fat; certain medications in the system, such as antihistamines; and the presence of a stomach enzyme called **dehydrogenase**, which helps to break down ethanol.

Alcohol dehydrogenase: any of various dehydrogenases [enzymes] that catalyze the reversible oxidation of an alcohol

When you drink, the alcohol that goes into your stomach and small intestine is absorbed by the bloodstream. It moves through membranes to the water in organs and other tissues, but little is absorbed by fat. Because women have proportionately more fat and relatively smaller quantities of blood than men, the same amount of alcohol will have a greater concentration in their bodies. Women may also have less stomach enzyme to decrease the level of ethanol before absorption. If they are pregnant, the alcohol is readily transported to the fetus through the blood-rich placenta.

Finally, the sugar in wine or mixed drinks adds to the dietary energy load of the body. If it isn't offset by taking in fewer calories or expending more calories through exercise, it will be converted to fat and cause weight gain.

How long does it take for the intoxicating effects of alcohol in the body to spike and then decline—or, in other words, how long does it take to "get a buzz" and to "sober up" after a drink?

According to the National Institutes of Health, "On an empty stomach, blood alcohol concentration peaks about one hour after consumption, depending on the amount drunk; it then declines in a more or less linear manner for the next four hours."[7]

Now you can understand how alcohol enters the body to affect the brain and spinal cord, the information superhighway of the central nervous system. Yes, drinking lets you relax and let down your guard, which can be fun and positive. At the same time, any level of impairment can alter your judgment, memory, balance, depth perception, muscle control, and so many other functions that maintain your equilibrium. That's why mental mistakes, accidental injury, and even death become more likely when people are under the influence of alcohol.

Before we run through those difficult scenarios, let's talk about why people enjoy drinking in the first place. What are the benefits to having a few beers with friends, drinking wine with a meal, or putting together a well-balanced cocktail? Does drinking make you happier? More creative? Healthier in any way? Let's find out.

---

7 Alex Paton, "Alcohol in the Body," *BMJ (Clinical research ed., 2005)*, 330(7482), 85–87, accessed June 6, 2020, https://doi.org/10.1136/bmj.330.7482.85.

The Upside of Alcohol

The benefits of drinking fall into two classes: emotional, and biologically based. They stem from the immediate physiological effects, which can be interpreted, in some cases, as either positive or negative. Over the years, these valuations have changed. Prior to 1800, for instance, religious leaders believed that God gave humans alcohol to use in moderation for their health and enjoyment. It was the abuse of alcohol, they thought, that was a sin. Nevertheless, people turned to excessive drinking as a mood enhancer and social lubricant. As industrialization progressed, though, and alcohol use threatened productivity and safety around machinery, those benefits were outweighed by its risks.

Today, we know more about the mechanisms of intoxication on the body. The pleasant ones include sedation and mild anesthesia, which help drinkers relax and overcome pain. Researchers believe alcohol triggers the "reward" centers of the brain with the release of dopamine and serotonin, the chemicals responsible for feelings of happiness. Drinkers report sensations of well-being, a lack of inhibition, and euphoria.

Feeling good makes folks more sociable, raising a sense

of camaraderie, unity, and shared purpose. This is why people make "toasts" with alcoholic beverages, play or watch sports over a few beers, or celebrate special events with a fine wine. These are the good times that many consider better when sharing a drink or two. And, how about creativity? Many artists, such as writer Ernest Hemingway and sculptor Frederic Remington, were known to be avid drinkers who considered alcohol a catalyst to their creative success. According to Sian Bellock, PhD, this may be because alcohol's effect on the brain shifts the ability to focus on some things and ignore others, which facilitates creative problem solving.[8] In other words, it helps them think outside the box.

But emotional effects are difficult to quantify and tie to a specific cause. Just as religious thinkers attributed alcohol's gifts to God, promoters of temperance found alcohol use the primary cause for societal ills. We think of modern medical research as the decider regarding alcohol's pluses and minuses, but even that is not as definitive as it could be. According to the Mayo Clinic:

---

8 Sian Bellock, "Alcohol Benefits the Creative Process," *Psychology Today*, updated April 4, 2012, accessed May 5, 202,; https://www.psychologytoday.com/us/blog/choke/201204/alcohol-benefits-the-creative-process.

Researchers know surprisingly little about the risks or benefits of moderate alcohol use in healthy adults. Almost all studies of lifestyle, including diet, exercise, caffeine, and alcohol, rely on patient recall and truthful reporting of one's habits over many years. These studies may indicate that two things may be associated with one another, but not necessarily that one causes the other. It may be that adults who are in good health engage in more social activities and enjoy moderate amounts of alcohol, but that the alcohol has nothing to do with making them healthier.[9]

What, then, has science found to be beneficial about drinking? **Moderation**, generally accepted to be one drink for women and two for men, is the key. And moderate drinking may:

- reduce the risk of developing and dying of heart disease
- reduce the risk of stroke

9 Mayo Clinic, "Alcohol Use, Weighing Risks and Benefits," updated October 26, 2019, accessed May 5, 2020, https://www.mayoclinic.org/healthy-lifestyle/ nutrition-and-healthy-eating/in-depth/alcohol/art-20044551.

- reduce the risk of developing diabetes

But, obviously that depends on what you're drinking and what your other health habits are. And the Mayo Clinic stresses that a causal link hasn't been conclusively established. If you're downing sugar-laden cocktails and the rest of your diet is high in sugar and carbohydrates (which break down to form simple sugars), then your diabetes risk will not be tempered by alcohol. If you're drinking a few ounces of red wine per day, some University of California researchers say the antioxidants and other compounds will protect your cardiovascular health, as well as reduce your risk for diabetes, cancer, and the effects of dementia.[10]

So, great: there may be biological boosts from a drink or two per day. There definitely are social benefits that come in the form of bonding and shared happiness. What else can you gain from drinking?

I would argue that education, practice, and developing a palate for alcoholic beverages contributes to lifelong learning.

---

10 Lynn Alley, *Wine Spectator*, "New Study Sheds More Light on Antioxidants in Red Wine," December 31, 2001, accessed June 2, 2020, https://www.winespectator.com/articles/new-study-sheds-more-light-on-antioxidants-in-red-wine-21137.

Look how many people pursue wine tasting and collecting as a hobby. With a history that stretches back millennia, there is plenty to satisfy one's curiosity. The nuances of wine making, how wine acts on taste receptors, and simply encountering the type of wine that you really like can keep you engaged for years on end. The same goes for beer, cider, and liquor. Becoming a true connoisseur—which literally means, "a knower"—is a satisfying activity that you can share with others.

Whatever your positive reasons for drinking, keep in mind that the goal is pleasure. Enjoying your favorite beverages in moderation does produce feelings of happiness and well-being. Enjoying alcohol in like company compounds its benefits. That may be why our go-to toast is, *Cheers!*

The Darker Side of Drinking

The title of this book contains the words "safe drinking" because the reality is that overindulging can literally kill you. Drinking alcohol when you are going to be driving or working with machinery can have fatal consequences for you, people you love, and innocent folks who happen to be in the wrong place at the wrong time. Simply drinking too much, too fast can overwhelm your metabolism and poison your bloodstream with alcohol. As with marksmanship, without responsible practices, your pursuit of pleasure may have the opposite effect—permanently.

But knowing more about the risks and dangers of alcohol isn't just a gloom-and-doom scare tactic. It's a preface to finding the safest way for you, personally, to drink. We've considered the benefits. Once you know the potential harmful effects, and the legal hot water you can get into, you'll be able to put your knowledge to work. The following chapters will walk your though legal details and tips for drinking safely, in moderation. If you don't drink, you'll want to be aware of the potential consequences if those around you do. Here are the hard facts about what can go wrong if you take a wrong turn:

» Drinking, driving, and age

- Any amount of alcohol increases the risk of crashes among teens as compared with older drivers.

- In the 2017 national Youth Risk Behavior Survey, 16.5% of high school students had ridden with a driver who had been drinking alcohol within the previous month. Among students who drove, 5.5% drove when they had been drinking alcohol during the 30 days before the survey.

- In 2017, 15% of drivers aged 16–20 involved in fatal motor vehicle crashes had a BAC of .08% or higher (a level that is illegal for adults aged 21 and older in all states, except Utah, which has a BAC limit of .05).
- In 2017, 58% of drivers aged 15–20 who were killed in motor vehicle crashes after drinking and driving were not wearing a seat belt (based on known restraint use).
- Among male drivers aged 15–20 who were involved in fatal crashes in 2017, 31% were speeding at the time of the crash and 20% had been drinking.[11]

So, underage drinking and driving is linked to less compliance with seat belt and speed limit laws, which exist to

---

11 Centers for Disease Control and Prevention, "Teen Drivers: Get the Facts," updated October 30, 2019, accessed May 7, 2020, https://www.cdc.gov/motorvehiclesafety/teen_drivers/teendrivers_factsheet.html.

protect drivers and passengers. Good to know. In Chapter 4, we'll get into the legal repercussions, *for which those simply riding along may be liable.*

» Immediate negative effects on the body

- An increase in blood pressure and release of hormones may produce flushing, sweating, and rapid heartbeat. Alcohol causes the kidneys to excrete more urine than normal.

- Alcohol's effect on the brain may lead to slurred speech, difficulty walking or performing other motor skills, and vomiting.

- The mental impairment that accompanies any amount of alcohol in the system raises the risk of injury. In driving simulation, for instance, bus drivers with a legal blood alcohol concentration perceived that they could drive their vehicles through spaces that were too narrow. At the current legal limit, the risk of a road accident more than doubles, and at twice that alcohol concentration, the risk is ten times greater.[12]

- Alcohol induces drowsiness, and at high concentration can cause a loss of consciousness, sometimes called blackouts. At that level of intoxication, abnormal heart rate, respiratory failure, or inhalation of vomit may occur. A fall may produce broken bones or head injuries. Even simply falling into a deep sleep induced by alcohol may cause nerve or musculoskeletal injuries.

- After effects, sometimes called hangovers, include fatigue, insomnia, nausea, and headache.[13]

Most of these negative effects are the result of overimbibing. Any amount of alcohol, though, can make it difficult to drive or perform other complicated tasks. Fortunately, there is one great motivation to be more cautious when drinking and to drink within limits: **self-preservation**.

---

12 Paton, ibid.

13 Adam C. Adler, MD, "General Anesthesia," Medscape, updated June 7, 2018, accessed May 7, 2020, https://emedicine.medscape.com/article/1271543-overview#a1.

» Long-term harmful effects on the body

- **Liver disease.**
- **Digestive problems**, including inflammation of the stomach lining and pancreas, as well as stomach and esophageal ulcers.
- **Heart problems** such as chronic high blood pressure, heart failure, or stroke.
- **Diabetes complications** such as hypoglycemia, which is dangerous to those who take insulin to reduce blood sugar levels.
- **Vitamin deficiency**, specifically vitamin B-1 (thiamin), which can lead to weakness and paralysis of eye muscles.
- **Bone damage**, causing a greater risk of fractures and reduced red blood cell production, which may result in bruising and bleeding.
- **Neurological complications** such as numbness and pain in hands and feet, disordered thinking, short-term memory loss and dementia.
- **Cancer** of the mouth, throat, liver, esophagus, colon, and breast. Even moderate drinking can

increase the risk of breast cancer.

- **Weakened immune system**, increasing the risk of infectious diseases, especially pneumonia.

- **Sexual function and menstruation issues**, including erectile dysfunction in men and menstruation disorders in women.

- **Birth defects** brought on by alcohol use during pregnancy may cause miscarriage or physical and developmental problems in the surviving child.[14]

These severe health problems may develop over time with regular or excessive alcohol use, depending on your personal medical history and other health habits. While they may seem remote now, the choices you make will determine drinking patterns that may persist for a lifetime. Alcohol is physically and/or psychologically habit-forming, meaning that frequent or high-volume drinkers can become dependent on it and find it difficult to quit.

Smoking is similarly addictive and potentially harmful.

---

14 Mayo Clinic, "Alcohol Use Disorder," updated July 11, 2018, accessed May 7, 2020, https://www.mayoclinic.org/diseases-conditions/alcohol-use-disorder/symptoms-causes/syc-20369243.

While young people are warned off of tobacco use with public service ads that show the long-term consequences, they may never see similar advice about alcohol use. Let this be your guidance now, so these health issues won't curtail your future.

Who Should Not Drink?

You may have moral or religious objections to drinking alcohol, or you simply may not find the practice interesting or enjoyable. Alcohol is considered an acquired taste, which is why young people are not encouraged to try it or to form habits too early. Due to ideology, biology, or even ethnicity, some people will never have positive experiences with alcohol. If you fall into one of these groups, drinking may not be for you.

The main physical reason to avoid drinking, apart from pregnancy, is generally a below-average alcohol tolerance. This typically results from low levels of stomach dehydrogenase. This is true of most Native North American Indians and some people of Asian heritage. Your family history should let you know whether you may have problems safely drinking alcohol.

Certain other people who should not drink, either temporarily or permanently, include those who are:

- planning on driving
- will be operating machinery
- pregnant
- unable to control the amount they drink

Additionally, don't drink if you are taking pain, anxiety, or other interactive medications. Be sure to read the labels on any medicine you take. And ask your doctor if you have a medical condition that can get worse with drinking, such as diabetes or heart problems.[15] No one but you can decide whether you will drink. If your body can't cope with intoxication, you won't enjoy it anyway. So, why risk your health?

Besides threats to health, drinking alcohol can have another huge impact on your life and your future. If you wind up with legal problems related to underage drinking or driving under the influence (DUI), your world could turn upside down. If you get someone else hurt or killed because you were impaired by alcohol, your life may never be the same. Going back to the parallels with marksmanship, enjoying alcoholic beverages is

15 MedlinePlus, "Alcohol," National Institutes of Health, U.S. National Library of Medicine, updated March 17, 2020, accessed May 7, 2020, https://medlineplus.gov/alcohol.html.

both a privilege and a responsibility. When you respect both of those caveats, you'll be on the road to safe drinking.

4

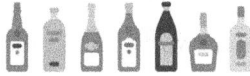

ALCOHOL AND THE LAW

How Unsafe Drinking Can Get You in Legal Hot Water

Safety is a must when using a potentially lethal substance. It also just happens to be a way to keep your driver's license, maintain a good insurance standing, and stay out of jail. Besides those preventive measures, safe drinking can save you money! Now I've got your attention; right?

Self-preservation is a powerful motivator. Not wanting to hurt or kill yourself is natural. Not wanting to harm others, while altruistic, is one more attitude that preserves your health and autonomy by preventing legal woes and damage to your future plans. Nobody wants to put themselves in a situation that might lead to fines, incarceration, or liability for someone else's injury or death. While you may be in a party mood when drinking, caution should always accompany that good feeling.

There are a host of legal considerations associated with drinking. These fall into two categories for newbies: laws about underage purchase, possession, intoxication, and driving; and laws for everyone else. We'll visit liability issues for injuring other people only briefly. Those are for the experts to explain. We will be concerned with all of the other things that can change your life, now and down the road. You may want to enjoy alcohol, but you also want to be in control of your present and future. That's good enough reason to stay in control of your drinking.

State and local jurisdictions dictate the nuances of alcoholic beverage regulation. It's up to citizens to inform themselves about the restrictions and consequences that apply where they live. I'll get you started here, but I suggest you do some more homework about the laws in your state and city or town. Ignorance of the law is never an excuse for breaking it. Don't even try that defense on police or judges! Or your parents, for that matter.

If you think it couldn't happen to you, here are some statistics ranging from 2010 to 2018.

- Approximately 10,000 people are killed in the U.S. each year in alcohol-impaired driving crashes, including drivers, passengers, pedestrians, and cyclists.

- Nearly one in five of those fatalities in 2010 were children through age 14 years. **More than half of all fatalities were passengers of vehicles with drivers who had BACs greater than or equal to 0.08%.** Men were responsible for 81 percent of these drunk-driving incidents.

- **Among major U.S. crimes, driving under the influence has one of the highest arrest rates**, with more than 1.4 million total DUI arrests in 2010.

- Drunk drivers may face jail time and the loss of their license and car when they're caught. **A DUI charge or conviction can cost as much as $10,000** in attorney's fees, fines, court costs, lost work wages, higher insurance rates, car towing, and more.

- Alcohol use can also impair boaters' judgment, balance, vision, and reaction time. The U.S. Coast Guard reported 154 recreational boating fatalities in which intoxication was a contributing factor in 2010.

- Excessive alcohol consumption increases aggression

and, as a result, can increase the risk of physically assaulting another person.

Here are a few statistics that are specific to underage drinking:

- Approximately 119,000 emergency rooms visits by persons aged 12 to 21 were for injuries and other conditions linked to alcohol in 2013.
- More than 1,000 people under 21 die every year in car crashes involving underage drinking.
- Teens who drink are more likely than nondrinkers to get into a car with a driver who has been drinking, smoking cannabis, using inhalants, or carrying a weapon.

(Sources: Federal Trade Commission; U.S. Department of Transportation; Bureau of Transportation Statistics; National Highway Traffic Safety Administration, Centers for Disease Control and Prevention, 2010–2018.)

As you can see from that last analysis by the CDC, **you don't have to be driving—or even drinking—to get into alcohol-related legal trouble.** Simply riding in a car with someone who is impaired can associate you with other crimes that they might commit, including drug possession and armed offenses. You may have to prove your innocence in court.

So, exactly what can cause legal trouble: by underage drinkers? by those of legal drinking age? And how might the laws change in the future to take the burden of secrecy and lawlessness off of people who are under 21? Let's find out.

Underage Drinking: What's Allowed, What's Penalized

While laws can change at any time, the drinking age of 21 set by federal law in 1984 currently holds for purchase and public possession of alcohol. But, guess what: **consumption on private property is permitted in a majority of states,** as shown on this map:

WHERE MINORS CAN LEGALLY DRINK IN THE U.S.

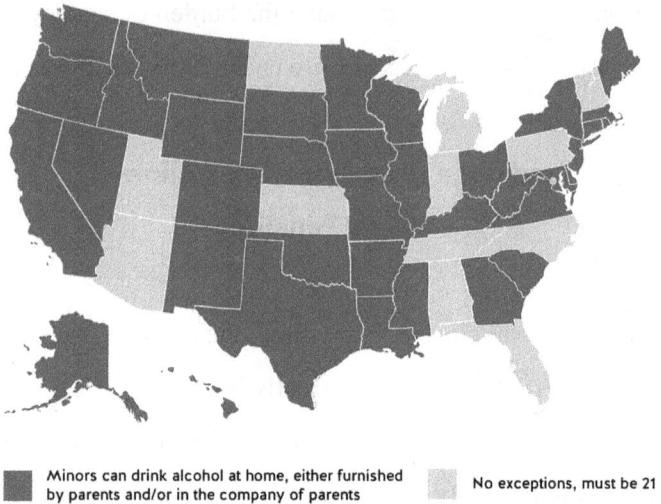

| | Minors can drink alcohol at home, either furnished by parents and/or in the company of parents | | No exceptions, must be 21 |

In addition, a few states allow minors accompanied by adults to drink in licensed restaurants and bars. Rather than summarize the confusing patchwork of statutes here, I'll ask you to review the current underage drinking policies in your home and bordering states at the National Institute on Alcohol Abuse and Alcoholism (NIAAA), which offers up-to-date information at https://alcoholpolicy.niaaa.nih.gov/underage-drinking/state-profiles. This website discloses whether it is illegal and if there are exceptions in your area:

- to possess or consume alcohol
- for adults to buy alcohol for minors
- to host underage drinking parties, regardless of the host's age

I can tell you, however, what the main types of permissions mean, if your state does have an exception to the federal law. These include allowances for whether people under age 21 can *possess* or *consume* alcohol, as well as legal allowances for parents, themselves, who want to provide alcohol to their children. Some regulations are based on religious or medical criteria, and others are based on adult distribution of alcohol or drinking supervision by a parent, guardian, or other person age 21 and up. Some exceptions specify whether drinking can occur indoors or out, and whether the private property must be a residence or not.

So, in some states, minors can drink alcoholic beverages provided by a parent or other adult without supervision, on private property. Some states require adult oversight. Laws in some places allow minors to possess but not consume alcohol— perhaps to allow them to give a bottle of wine bought by an adult to another adult. You might actually need an attorney's opinion to sort all this out, but the NIAAA website will give you a starting point for what you need to know.

Nowhere in the United States can those under 21 use false identification to purchase alcohol. While a few states (Delaware, Indiana, New York, and Vermont) don't outright prohibit purchase by minors, they do prohibit consumption! If you are under 21 and caught buying, possessing, or drinking in illegal situations, there are additional laws regarding evidence of your guilt, should your case go to court: certain jurisdictions need proof of possession, such as a bottle. Some require proof of *internal possession;* in other words, test results that the minor had alcohol in their system. Others want proof of consumption, like an eye-witness account or admission of guilt by the minor—and possibly a combination of these types of evidence.

As you can see, simply drinking alcohol responsibly is not the limit of your obligation under the law. Add the restrictions on driving and providing alcohol to other minors, and the legal landmines really add up. So do the penalties, if you're a repeat offender. Here are a few penalties for offenses related to underage drinking that exist in various states:[16]

» Buying alcohol with a fake id

- confiscation of ID
- detention by the retailer until authorities arrive
- if charged, fines, jail time, community service probation, and suspension of driving privileges may apply
- retailers can sue the minor for up to $1000 in damages

» Purchasing, possessing, or consuming alcohol as a minor

- confiscation of alcohol
- driver's license suspension for 30 to 730 days
- driver's license revocation for 30 to 730 days, after which the offender must reapply for a license
- fines of $250 to $500
- 24 to 48 hours of compulsory community service

16 American Addiction Centers, "Underage Drinking," updated 2020, accessed May 12, 2020, https://www.projectknow.com/discover/under-age-drinking/.

If your alcohol offense is combined with driving, you may face fines, jail time, and/or mandatory alcohol abuse counseling, as well as lose your insurance coverage and even your vehicle, temporarily. Furthermore, if you injure or kill someone due to impaired driving, your criminal and civil liability can mean major prison time and sky-high monetary judgments. And, you're not the only one who can get in trouble by drinking underage. If you do buy alcohol in a state where it is prohibited, the retailer can get socked with a fine as high as $10,000. An adult who buys for you can get a steep fine and up to a year's jail time.

It's easy to say, *Think about these things before you decide to drink.* It's up to you to actually do it.

Of-Age Consequences

If you're over 21, you can legally drink at home, on other people's properties, and in licensed restaurants and bars. **You can't supply alcohol to minors**, unless you fall under one of the exceptions for parents, guardians, or spouses that may exist in your locale. Doing so may result in a thousand-dollar fine and compulsory community service. If you overserve drinkers of any age on your own property (causing them to exceed the legal BAC limit), you can be held liable if they hurt someone because they are intoxicated. This is called **social host liability,** which may embroil you in an expensive lawsuit.

Do you drive? Every state has a legal blood-alcohol intoxication limit for drivers, usually 0.08%, but not every state outright prohibits drinking *while* driving, up to that limit. On the other hand, in some states, you can get arrested just for having open containers of alcohol in the car. Police stops at DUI checkpoints can leave you open to searches and breathalyzer tests to determine whether or not you are in violation of state laws.

Again, you'll have to research your own area's regulations. Your state motor vehicle division website will have a link to that information. Here, I'd like to talk about the potential consequences of driving under the influence in terms that everyone can understand: financial and legal. In other words, **what might a DUI charge or conviction cost in terms of your wallet and your freedom?**

Let's look at a hypothetical DUI situation in, say, California. Under current state law, what might happen?

If you're pulled over and an officer suspects you may be intoxicated, you're required to give a blood or breath test. If you refuse, you'll be fined $125 and your license will be suspended for a year.

If you test above the legal BAC of 0.08%, your driver's license may be confiscated, your car towed and impounded, and you may be arrested and detained—though probably released within 24 hours—pending a court hearing.

If you are convicted in court, some or all of these penalties may apply:

- License suspension, 4 to 10 months
- Use of vehicle interlock ignition device (IID) for 6 months after license reinstatement (IID is a breathalyzer that won't allow your car to start unless it tests you to be alcohol-free)
- Fines from $390 to $1000, or more
- Probation or jail time, 2 days to 6 months
- Probation includes 30 hours of DUI school, which

costs about $600

- If you injure or kill someone in relation to your DUI offense, criminal fines may reach $5000 and prison time can range from 1 year to life

In addition, you might have to pay car towing, impound, and attorney's fees. You might lose time from work, or even lose your job. If you hit another car and cause personal injury or death, you might be sued for hundreds of thousands of dollars or more. Getting pulled over and grilled by a traffic cop will be the least of your worries. **So, don't drink and drive!** That has a little broader meaning now; doesn't it?

Potential Changes

The legal drinking age of 21 lies at the root of problems related to young people and drinking. But it doesn't have to stay that way. Why might the U.S. change federal or state drinking laws? After reading this chapter, you'll probably agree: because they are inconsistent. They're inconsistent from state to state, inconsistent with the reality that young people drink, and inconsistent with the supposed goal of keeping youth drinkers safe.

Pressuring young people into lawlessness or ignorance is risky, not safe.

As I've mentioned, forcing teenagers into the shadows to satisfy the urge to experiment with alcohol removes them from any beneficial adult oversight. They may wind up binge drinking, driving to a place where they can drink, or simply drinking unsafely because they don't understand their limits or the health consequences. As Dr. David J. Hanson, an expert on alcohol policy and a professor of sociology at State University of New York Potsdam, relates, our confusing patchwork of laws does not deliver a clear message on how to enter the drinking public. Instead, "they reflect the fact that we as a society don't really agree on how to deal with alcohol."

But it is our duty to create fair and consistent laws, not to confuse people into running afoul of them. While ignorance of statutes isn't a viable excuse for breaking them, misunderstanding your legal obligations means that you can violate laws without knowing it. You can even be found guilty of infractions that didn't occur simply because evidence suggests it did—such as someone else's empty bottle being found in your car. "I suspect many people are being convicted for crimes they didn't commit because of the confusion," Dr. Hanson admits.

This situation is reflected in the conflicting popular views of alcohol that prevail, in both marketing and personal standards. When ads equate beer drinking with endless parties, and yet one in every seven adults claims drinking is a sin,[17] what are young people to conclude? The fact is, they reach their own conclusions, usually based on scant information and little practical experience.

Suppose the drinking age were lowered to better conform to reality: the age when people can safely start drinking, prefaced by unbiased education. The latter could be tied to the former. It might work the way graduated driver's licenses do. You'd take a class, get a permit, have a probationary period, and gain full rights to drink responsibly. There are many ways to change the structure of federal and state drinking laws. For some guidelines, let's consider how other countries differ from the U.S. in regulating the sale and use of alcohol, particularly the age and supervision factors.

First, let's look at the importance of adult guidance. If we accept that training of the uninitiated by experienced people—in any situation—is a good thing, it's easy to see how supervised

---

17 Ingraham, ibid.

drinking can help those who are new to the practice. Consider an apprentice learning to design and make a violin. These skills could be learned from a book or trial-and-error alone. But they could likely be mastered much more quickly and with greater insight with the help of an expert. So it goes with learning to safely enjoy alcohol.

A Canadian study published in the *Journal of Drug and Alcohol Dependence* found that **44 percent of teenage drinkers overall experience negative alcohol-related incidents, such as injury or overdose.** Those who received alcohol from their parents versus from their friends, however, reported fewer alcohol-related harms.[18] This suggests that parents' "condoning" drinking does not increase problem behavior. In fact, it normalizes alcohol consumption and may reduce the risk of abuse later in life.

Furthermore, the findings of a U.S. study published in the *Journal of Adolescent Health* pointed toward parental *supervision* as a restraining factor in risky drinking habits. A

---

18 M.N. Wilson, et al. "When Parents Supply Alcohol to Their Children: Exploring Associations with Drinking Frequency, Alcohol-related Harms, and the Role of Parental Monitoring," PMID: 29248692. DOI: 10.1016/j. drugalcdep.2017.10.037; accessed May 13, 2020, https://www.ncbi.nlm. nih.gov/pubmed/29248692.

wide sample of more than six thousand teenagers who reported drinking an occasional glass of wine with parents were 66 percent less likely to binge-drink with friends.[19] Could it be because "apprenticeship" allows less experienced drinkers to learn responsible practices from people whom they know and trust?

Now, let's examine how other countries handle introducing young people to alcohol. Familial drinking is far more widespread in nations such as France, Italy, and the United Kingdom, and thus, children learn moderation by example from an early age. This may be why the legal drinking age is typically lower outside the U.S. The National Highway Traffic Safety Administration notes, "Interestingly, in most countries the minimum age for driving licensure is older than or equal to the drinking age, unlike the United States, in which all states allow licensure well before drinking is permitted."[20]

That seems much more reasonable than prohibiting behavior that already occurs at a young age. Many countries around

19 Kristie Long Foley, et al., "Adults' Approval and Adolescents' Alcohol Use," J Adolesc Health, 2004 Oct;35(4):345.e17-26, accessed 13 May 13, 2020, https://pubmed.ncbi.nlm.nih.gov/15830441/.

20 National Highway Traffic Safety Administration, "On DWI Laws in Other Countries," March 2000, accessed May 13, 2020, https://one.nhtsa.gov/people/injury/research/pub/DWIothercountries/dwiothercountries.html.

the world, including England, Brazil, and Australia, set the drinking and driving ages at 18. Switzerland allows beer and wine consumption at age 14 and liquor at age 18. Others fall somewhere in between. This allows law enforcement to tie drinking privileges to driving privileges—something that U.S states already do, but while still upholding abstinence rather than consumption within legal limits. Again, **when forced to circumvent the law, young people must also circumvent parental and other adult supervision**.

Instead, young drinkers could be guided under the "apprenticeships" of bar and restaurant servers, retailers, teachers, and, of course, parents. Given the recent reform of other laws concerning controlled substances, the laws on when Americans can legally imbibe may well change. It's important for those who choose to drink—just like those who choose to drive or choose to use a gun—to monitor the laws that govern their behavior.

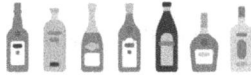

5

SAFE (AND UNSAFE) DRINKING PRACTICES

Tips to Moderate and Mellow the Effects of Drinking

And now, the moment you've been waiting for: practical ideas on how you can enhance the upside and reduce the downside of alcohol use. After all, enjoyment and good health are the goals. How many ways are there to toast to that effect? *¡Salud! À santé! To your health!*

Some positive drinking behavior comes in response to what you *don't* want to happen—those "alcohol-related harms" the scientists talk about. So, these tips are meant to head off problems, particularly those related to getting dehydrated, becoming dependent on alcohol, losing control of your mental and physical functions, and getting too much sugar in your diet. If you prevent those problems, you'll prevent others that are associated with them.

But we've had enough of the tough consequences you might face for now. We'll get to the "wrong" way to drink, and why it's wrong, later in this chapter. In the following chapter, we'll talk more about calculating your alcohol intake limit to safeguard your future health, and learning more about the beverages you find most interesting. For now, let's take advantage of what humans have learned over millennia of imbibing for pleasure. It's a relatively short list of "do's" that you can keep in your toolbox and lend to others.

Tips on How to Drink Safely

1. **Drink enough water every day.** If you start out well hydrated, it will take longer for the ethanol concentration to build up. How much water? For men, about 13 cups. For women, about 9 cups.

   - **Recommended Daily Water Intake (1 cup = 8 ounces:**

Men: 13 cups (104 ounces, about 3 liters)

Women: 9 cups (72 ounces, about 2 liters)

2. **Know your drink limit and decide how you'll stick with it.** This will depend on what kind of alcohol you're drinking, whether it's mixed with anything, and how your personal condition may alter the standard limit of one to two drinks for women and two to three for men. Read the labels and do some extra research online if you need to determine how much alcohol you'll be getting per drink. We'll do the math on limits in Chapter 6.

   • **Standard Drink Limit:**

     Men: 2 to 3 drinks

     Women: 1 to 2 drinks

3. **Plan ahead for transportation home.** Designate a driver, know your walking route, or plan on public transportation so you won't be tempted to drink and drive. If you do drive and overimbibe, don't be afraid to get a taxi, use a rideshare app, or call home and ask for a ride by a sober driver.

4. **Invest in a personal breathalyzer.** This takes the

guesswork out of when to stop drinking or whether you should be driving.

5. **Factor in any medications you've taken.** Many drugs shouldn't be combined with alcohol. If you don't have medicine labels handy, don't drink.

6. **Don't drink on an empty stomach.** Eat something beforehand and while you drink. Foods with protein such as eggs, cheese, or unsalted nuts are good choices. Snacks with high vitamin, mineral, and water content— including bananas, berries, and melon—are good too.

7. **Sip, don't gulp.** It's not a race, since moderation is the goal. Think quality, not quantity. You'll enjoy your drink more, and it will last longer.

8. **Alternate between alcoholic beverages and water, not soda pop.** If you're having more than one drink, you can savor them over time by having a glass of water in between and afterwards. You'll already get enough sugar in any beverage alcohol or mixers, and zero calories is a nice number.

9. **Respect those who don't want to drink or who have had enough.** Never insist that friends "just try a sip" or have "one for the road." Drinking is complicated enough

without undue pressure.

10. **Say no when you've had enough.** It can be tempting when a server asks if you'd like one more or someone buys a round of drinks for the table. Remember that those are *their* actions, not yours. You don't have to drink just because it is offered.

11. **Never accept a drink from someone you don't know.** Just say, "No, thanks," or give your order to the server— and watch the bartender make the drink. It's your right to know what you're drinking.

12. **Don't play drinking games.** These are geared toward overindulgence and raise the risk of getting sick or passing out. Watch and cheer if you must, but don't play. Drinking is not a game.

Unsafe Scenarios to Avoid

1. **Too many drinks in a short time.** "Slamming" drinks, playing games like Quarters or Beer Pong, or just guzzling as fast as you can raises your blood alcohol level rapidly. This type of excess, or binge drinking, greatly increases your risk for injury, car wrecks, and

alcohol poisoning. It can also trigger aggression and leave you subject to liability if you injure someone or vulnerable to violence by others.

- **What Is Alcohol Poisoning?** Alcohol poisoning can occur when a person drinks large quantities of alcohol, including beer, wine, and liquor, in a relatively short time. As the amount of alcohol in the bloodstream increases, the liver can't break down the alcohol and remove its toxins from the blood quickly enough.

    The excess alcohol acts as a depressant and causes parts of the brain that control vital body functions–including breathing, heart rate, blood pressure, and temperature–to shut down. The blood alcohol content (BAC) can continue to rise 40 minutes after the last drink, as alcohol in the stomach and intestines continues to enter the bloodstream. Source: Cleveland Clinic.

2. **Too many drinks over a long period of time.** Alcohol can be habit forming, and the resulting alcoholism degrades your health and increases your risk for financial, legal, and social trouble. You don't need to make

drinking routine, especially if you are young or new to alcohol. Make a conscious effort to change up how often or how much you drink, and to take weeks or months off from drinking.

3. **Drinking during the day.** Some people drink when they wake up to "cure" a hangover, but starting early gives you a potential window for excess. It may also indicate a growing problem with depression or an inability to control your drinking.

4. **Mixing alcohol and sex.** Consent and preventing pregnancy are two important facets of responsible sexual activity. Alcohol impairs your judgment on both counts and may have dire consequences. Being drunk is no excuse for unprotected sex and no substitute for consensual sex.

5. **Mixing alcohol and drugs.** Prescription medications and controlled substances only add to your level of alcohol impairment and all of the risks we've talked about.

6. **Drinking and driving or boating.** States impose steep penalties for operating all types of watercraft and motor vehicles, for good reason. Driving or boating

while intoxicated puts yourself and those around you in harm's way.

7. **Drinking and operating machinery.** Whether you use machines at work or at home, doing so while impaired increases your chance of injury or death. Something as simple as mowing a lawn can lead to a tragic accident if you misjudge what you can safely do with sharp blades, gasoline, or electrical cords.

8. **Drinking until you pass out.** Blacking out from intoxication may seem benign, but losing consciousness is not the same as drifting off to sleep. Passing out can affect your memory, breathing, body posture, and ability to get help if you need it. You could be held liable for actions that you don't recall, inhale vomit due to blocked airways, suffer nerve or musculoskeletal damage, or even die from untreated alcohol poisoning.

9. **Sleeping under the influence.** Even if you don't involuntarily lose consciousness, sleeping while drunk creates a state of "depressed consciousness," which may disrupt normal bodily functions. Certainly you might fail to hear a smoke alarm or other warning in the event of fire or another emergency. Besides the possibility of

winding up in the wrong position for a period long enough to cause muscle or nerve damage, your ability to swallow and breathe may also be compromised. In this state, if you've drunk enough to make you sick, you might vomit, swallow, and breathe in quick succession, meaning you'll draw stomach contents into your lungs. This can kill you, as it has in many high-profile cases of celebrities, including Elvis Presley, Jimi Hendrix, John Bonham, Bon Scott, and Amy Winehouse. "Don't drink and sleep" may be just as dire a commandment as "don't drink and drive."

10. **Drinking if you are pregnant.** You'll find warnings against this selfish practice on every container of alcoholic beverage sold in America, so no one can claim ignorance of its dangers. Mothers who drink can develop high blood pressure, experience miscarriage or premature birth, and cause birth defects that may adversely affect the child for life.

These are avoidable situations. You don't have to make the same errors that other people have, in many cases simply because they didn't know any better. I always say, it's good to learn from the mistakes of others! Remember, we're not examining these risks to tell you not to drink, but to allow you to drink in moderation and for fun and enjoyment, when the time is right for you. If you're lucky enough to be reading this before trying alcoholic beverages, you can feel good about being able to make informed decisions based on the facts—not on societal or peer pressure.

6

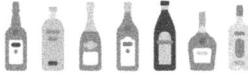

ALCOHOL AND YOUR FUTURE

Where Will You Go from Here?

When you start drinking as a youth or later in life, the closest you may get to imagining your future with alcoholic beverages is to look forward to a Friday-night drink on the deck. In this chapter, we'll attempt to broaden your horizons to envision which aspects of social drinking you might like to pursue. Learning more about craft brewing, winemaking, or how to make fancy cocktails can be terrific hobbies. To actually do those things, though, you'll have to stay healthy in the near term and avoid chronic health problems in the long term. Let's visit those topics one more time, in order to set you up for success.

Watch Your Calories

Whether you're concerned about your weight now or not, you will be as you grow older. Habitually consume food or beverages with "empty" calories—energy with fewer vitamins and minerals than more nutritionally dense foods or drinks—makes it easy to put on pounds over the years and not take them off. The typical American diet is high in sugar and carbohydrates, which become body fat if their calories are not worked off. And, according to the CDC, 42 percent of Americans are obese, or seriously overweight. To keep alcohol a positive element in your life, you'll want to watch the calories , which is easiest to do if you drink in moderation.

Obesity is not a fun condition itself, but it is also a risk factor in many chronic, or long-term, diseases, including:

- cancer
- heart disease
- stroke
- type 2 diabetes

Your chances for developing this last one are heightened by drinking alcohol, because many alcoholic beverages contain sugar. High intake of added sugars is a known contributor to diabetes. This chronic disease can have deadly side effects, and it may require you to curtail your diet or take expensive insulin medication for the rest of your life.

I draw your attention to this because certain beverages that are popular with young drinkers—maybe because they are purposely marketed to this demographic—have excessive sugar content. Dietary guidelines suggest limiting total dietary sugar to 38 grams per day for men and 25 grams per day for women. (They also suggest getting just 10% of your total calories from sugar; but for our purposes, if you're limiting drink calories, you're limiting sugar intake.) The carb or sugar content of brand-name ready-to-drink cocktails that I researched, for instance, ranged from 26 to 40 grams per serving. That's a full day's allowance ... and that's if you only drink one, not counting the other sugar in your diet. If you had a piece of cake, for instance, that's 15 grams of sugar, plus the calorie count.

Even commercial drinks that aren't high in added sugar may taste sweet and not like alcohol at all, making you want to drink more of them. Bottled hard ciders, for instance, are yummy but may have greater calorie and carbohydrate content than beer. Remember, carbs break down into sugar during digestion ... and calories add up. Bring this to mind the next time you consider multiple drinks or super-sizing: restaurants and bars may offer 12-, 16-, or even 22-ounce draft beers, and the standard drink is based on 12 ounces. Factor total amounts into your personal alcohol-limit calculations. That's what we'll talk about next.

Recognize Your Drink Limits

Before you start your math, consider whether you have a special need to limit or abstain from alcohol. Are you:

- pregnant?
- Native American?
- of Asian descent?
- recovering from alcohol dependence?
- in a family with a history of alcoholism?
- on medications that might interact with alcohol?

If so, ask your doctor about whether or how much alcohol you can safely drink. You may want to do this anyway, to get started with confidence, on the right foot.

Otherwise, you can stick to the "one drink for women, two drinks for men" recommendation. But, if you're not driving and you are eating and staying hydrated, you might want to drink more. You could simply buy a personal breathalyzer and monitor yourself as you drink and afterwards, as the alcohol is removed from the blood and processed by the liver, or metabolized. This lag time is the amount of time it takes for you to "burn off" alcohol or for a drink to "wear off."

You could also use a formula devised by a Swedish researcher named Erik Widmark that ties those physical functions to metrics related to gender, how much you drink, and how strong the drinks are. When you multiply the number of standard drinks by a constant that averages metabolic time (3.5 for men, 4.7 for women) and then divide by your weight, you'll arrive at a general BAC.

BAC Using the Widmark Formula

Example 1: A 120-pound woman drinks 2 tequila shots.

2 x 4.7 = 9.4

9.4 / 120 = .08 BAC

Example 2: A 180-pound man drinks 4 beers.

4 x 3.75 = 15

15/ 180 = .08 BAC

For a quick calculation, you can use an online tool created by the Cleveland Clinic based on this formula. **To get a ballpark estimate, record:**

- your weight
- size of beverage in ounces
- its percentage of alcohol content (abv)
- how long you plan to be drinking

Source: http://www.clevelandclinic.org/health/interactive/alcohol_calculator.asp.

Both examples in the box result in a BAC that is about the 0.08% legal limit. **Suppose you go over that limit. When would it be safe to drive?** That entails more math. Alcohol in the blood is eliminated, or drops, at a rate of about 0.02 BAC per hour. So, if you were at 0.10% and waited an hour, your BAC would drop to about 0.08%. Contrary to popular myth, drinking coffee won't sober you up. Neither will drinking water, although that does keep you from becoming dangerously dehydrated from alcohol. Only the passage of time allows your liver and kidneys to remove alcohol from your system.

Which of these actions will sober you up?

a. Waiting for the ethanol in your bloodstream to be removed by the liver and kidneys

b. Drinking one or more glasses of water

c. Drinking a cup of coffee

(Answer: a.)

What does this mean for your personal drinking boundaries? You'll learn to identify them over time, but it pays to be aware. Consider how you feel: after one, two, or more drinks. Consider how those affect your reaction time, speech, balance, mental judgment, et cetera. You might even jot these things down. What seems to be your best alcohol intake? What makes you feel good—perhaps pleasantly buzzed, but not off-kilter? When have you overdone it? These things vary from person to person, but the legal BAC limit for driving will be fixed. You'll need to accommodate both of those boundaries, if you drive and if you want to stay healthy over time.

Develop Your Palate

Are you ready for happy hour? Armed with the facts and tools to manage your use of alcohol, you can sit back and enjoy it. But, what suits your tastes? These days, with the advent of micro and craft breweries and distilleries, new winemaking practices, and ingenious new cocktail formulas, there are more options than ever. You might start out by touring a winery, brewery, or distillery to get the inside story, firsthand. Here are a few roads you might travel to arrive at your "happy place."

Craft beers and ciders. Are you a numbers person? Craft brewing gives you exact scientific measurements of the various elements in beer, ale, and cider. These include color (from pale to black, defined by a chart called standard reference method, or SRM); level of bitterness (which comes from hops content, gauged in international bitterness units, or IBU); and alcohol by volume, which you already know as ABV. When you learn what you like in flavor and strength, you'll be able to compare different brews by these numbers, which many brewpubs list on their menus.

Winemaking and wine tasting. Both are fascinating processes. Delve into how grapes are grown, harvested, and sourced. Learn about the different wine-growing regions, or appellations, in the United States and around the world. Get to know the language of wine tasting, which likens the various flavor elements to other well-known tastes, such as: fruits, flowers, spices, smoke, and earth. As you practice tasting wine, you'll notice the difference in flavor and color from year to year, and whether you prefer wines that are sweet, dry, straight-forward, or complex. Wineries typically offer visitors "tasting flights," a series of pours drawn from different varietals, vintages, and bottlings.

Trends in spirits. For decades, established distilleries—such as makers of traditional Kentucky bourbon and imported scotch and vodka—had a lock on the production and sale of liquor, but no more. Local distilleries have opened up the market for craft spirits. You'll find small-batch gins, vodkas infused with herbs or fruit, award-winning bourbons *not* made in Kentucky, and on and on. Producers are happy to promote the unique characteristics that set their spirits apart from the usual name brands. It's easy to get acquainted with the new liquor offerings by visiting a bar that carries local or unusual brands. Just ask the bartender what's popular and give it a try, straight or in a cocktail.

Seasonal drinks. Hot drinks in winter and blender drinks in summer expand the variety of cocktails you might enjoy. Cold-weather favorites like mulled wine, hot buttered rum, and alcoholic coffee drinks make winding down from winter sports or curling up near a fire more festive. Summertime spritzers that increase the volume of seltzer or fruit juice in wine or liquor cocktails are refreshing and allow you to sip longer and more leisurely. Additions from the garden, such as fresh mint, lavender, or rosemary make drinking in season special—especially outdoors, on a warm summer evening.

Presentation. Are you interested in which glass goes with which wine, and why? Do you love the little extras, like garnishes in cocktails, fancy corkscrews, or flaming drinks like Spanish coffees? Once you know what you like to drink, you can focus on *how* you like to drink. For instance, a Bloody Mary (vodka and tomato juice) loaded with celery, dill pickle, green olives, pickled green beans, and even bacon (yes, bacon!) makes an impressive presentation. Sometimes, just a fancy cocktail napkin or one printed with a theme illustration or funny joke will elevate a simple beverage to one that is meaningful in the moment. Drink accessories are a great way to turn happy hour into a bonding experience for friends and family.

You have now graduated from this instruction manual to your own "apprenticeship" in drinking drink safely and enjoyably. Congratulate yourself! You're ready to make choices on a much more sound basis than the vast majority of folks. And you're prepared to set off on what might be a lifelong journey of learning, camaraderie, and fun. Best of all, you are in a position to counsel others—those younger or less experienced than yourself, and more seasoned drinkers who may have missed out on this type of basic education.

This state of awareness and preparedness reminds me of

my early years, hunting with family. There is something about shared experience, in the moment, unique to the time and place that cannot be matched or duplicated. Making memories is satisfying that way. I wish you a long life of such moments, with the confidence that knowledge and self-determination brings. I wish you the best. *Cheers!*

A NOTE TO PARENTS AND TEACHERS

Why teach students—particularly those under the legal drinking age—about alcohol? Because, practically speaking, education is far more useful to them than prohibition. You don't have to drink a drop to need to know the facts about alcohol. Here are half a dozen reasons why:

- If you want young people to abstain, it's best to inform them of the dangers so they can own their choice not to drink and tell other people why.
- Nondrinkers may one day need to know how to recognize intoxication and what to do to help someone who has had too much to drink. This may save lives.
- People who are new to drinking must understand the mechanisms of how alcohol affects the body and mind. From this, they can recognize the value of drinking in moderation, rather than just being told to limit their drinking.
- Many of today's alcoholic beverages taste like soda pop,

not alcohol. Informing people about the sugar and alcohol content will remind them to treat these beverages with care.

- Not all alcoholic beverages are fully labeled the way food products are. Understanding how to read a label and how to find information that is not on the label is an important part of making safe choices.
- Early education is the foundation for decisions that affect a person's future.

www.ingramcontent.com/pod-product-compliance
Lightning Source LLC
Chambersburg PA
CBHW072151020426
42334CB00018B/1956